TOTAL FREEDOM FROM BODY ODOR

The Ultimate Professional Guide to Breaking Free From Body Odor

"Your Simplified Self-Help Book"

By

Dr. Suman Hashmi Das

TABLE OF CONTENT

CHAPTER ONE

A BRIEF ACCOUNT OF BODY ODOR

Although humans have always had a peculiar smell, over the ages, our understanding of what is "clean" has evolved significantly.

We take it for granted that being odorless equates to cleanliness in today's heavily deodorized society. But in all of humanity's long and fragrant history, smelling "good" has occasionally been repulsive as well as delightful.

You have to start with sweat if you must get to the root of body odor; however, the scent of human perspiration alone usually isn't very strong. According to writer Sarah Everts, who has studied the science of sweating extensively, "the problem is that bacteria living on our body like to eat some of the compounds that come out in our sweat." Both apocrine and eccrine glands, which are primarily located in the genital and armpit regions of the body, secrete a variety of substances that are eaten by bacteria and release molecules that give off the distinct odor that is known as body odor.

Naturally, for the majority of recorded history, humans were ignorant of this compound which is why the first attempts to smell civilized involved masking the unpleasant smells with more agreeable ones. "The ancient Egyptians applied concoctions made of ostrich eggs, tortoiseshell, and gallnuts to help improve their personal body pong," Everts explains. During this period, thick pastes or oil-based salves containing ingredients from aromatic plants such as cardamom, cassia, cinnamon, lemongrass, lily, myrrh, and rose were commonly worn as fragrances on the head, neck, and wrists.

Moreover, Egyptians invented jewelry with scented materials and burned fragrant incense—a custom that is still followed by societies in northern Africa. It is thought that the tiny cones that men and women wear atop their wigs in hieroglyphics were created from animal fats and scented wax. A popular luxury item in ancient Greece and Rome, fragrant spices and perfumes spread along trade routes connecting the Mediterranean and the Middle East. The Roman Empire, a unique historical era when taking a daily bath was common practice for both social and religious reasons, is when the earliest perfumeries are said to have existed. After soaking, the body was usually anointed with fragrant oils, which were occasionally carried in tiny bottles that were fastened to the wrist.

The floral scents of jasmine, rose, iris, lavender, violet, or chamomile were combined with spicy scents from natural ingredients like cloves, camphor, and yellow amber in the early creations of fragrances. Perfumes derived from animals included civet (from civet cats), musk (found in musk deer), or ambergris (a secretion of the sperm whale). Perfume-infused fabrics were used to sew clothing, and talc-based scented powders were transported in fabric sachets.

Incense and fragrant oils had permeated religious rites in Europe by the fifth century A.D., influencing both Christian and Jewish practices. Everyone brought their own unique scents to public worship areas because different social classes congregated there, and incense helped to cover up the stench of fear of God. "Priests were so overwhelmed by the stench of their worshipers that they would avidly burn incense to counteract the worshipers' body odor," Everts relates. The clergy occasionally mocked perfume as a sinful indulgence, even as they exalted religious incense. Due to its association with the sin of pride or vanity, bathing was frowned upon by many Christians for a number of centuries.

Islamic communities continued the tradition of bathing, while Christians preferred not to. Turkish baths, or hammams, originated from Roman bathing practices in the eastern Byzantine Empire. The custom of using hammas was revived in Europe in the eleventh century when Crusaders returned, bringing with them aromatic goods like civet and musk. Most soap at the time were harsh and smelled like the ash and animal fats they were made of, so people hardly ever used them on their skin. However, soap manufacturing replaced perfumes as the main use for perfumes after Middle Eastern innovators created improved formulas containing vegetable oils.

Chemists had perfected the process of distilling by the 13th century, which involves boiling a natural substance in water to extract its essential oil. These essential oils were mixed with alcohol by innovators to produce the modern, stable, and rapidly drying perfume. A late 14th-century rosemary perfume known as Hungary water—so named because it was created for Queen Elisabeth of

Hungary—was the first significant alcohol-based fragrance. The bubonic plague killed over a third of Europe's population and forced the closure of most public bathhouses. People used to think that diseases like the plague could spread through the air because of their lack of scientific understanding of germs.

This way, the sweet aroma of aromatics combated the sickly stink. "Specific diseases, like plague, believed to be conveyed by impure or corrupt air, were frequently countered by building bonfires in public spaces, and in private by burning incense or inhaling perfumes such as rose and musk," says Jonathan Reinarz, a professor of medical history who published a book called Past Scents: Historical Perspectives on Smell. As a common accessory to carry to cover the stench of death, little bouquets of flowers and herbs known as posies, nosegays, or tussie-mussies emerged.

Better hygiene through hand washing and bathing, however, is the real counter-measure to major epidemics, but it was out of reach as long as the majority of Europeans thought bathing posed a health risk. The myth that water's capacity to open pores and soften skin actually weakened the flesh was propagated in the 15th and 16th centuries by well-known scientists. Because of this, the few individuals who did take regular baths took extra care, such as applying oil to their bodies and covering themselves in scented cloths. Strong-smelling powders could be used to massage hair, and chewing on strong-smelling herbs could help with bad breath.

France started to take the lead in the global perfume market as more sophisticated floral or herbal scents became popular. One of its most well-known scents was eau de cologne, a concoction of citrus and rosemary essences suspended in a grape-based spirit that was first created as a plague remedy. The French nobility advanced the art of perfumery in the 17th and 18th centuries by creating their own unique essences and erecting fragrant fountains at their dinner parties. Neroli, an orange blossom scent, was added to leather gloves, which became one of the most popular products in the nation.

Tiny perfume boxes that were made to hold liquid perfumes quickly became the hottest accessory. These ornately perforated cases, also known as "smelling boxes," "pouncet boxes," and, subsequently, "vinaigrettes," contained tiny sponges or fabric swatches soaked in fragrances made of alcohol or vinegar that were praised for their medicinal properties as well as their ability to block out offensive odors from city streets. However, wealthy people frequently still stank even with access to perfumes. "Descriptions of Versailles by a lot of people visiting the court of Louis XVI and his bride, Marie Antoinette, just before the revolution are really striking," Reinarz claims. "They described it as a stinking cesspit."

The French Revolution saw a shift in fashion toward lighter cotton fabrics that were also easier to wash, simpler silhouettes, and fewer layers. Finally, bathing had become fashionable again, with medical professionals now holding the view that built-up dirt stopped the body from expelling tainted fluids. The mid-1800s saw cholera outbreaks that prompted cities all over Europe to build new sewer systems, increase fresh water availability, and organize waste disposal. The industry aligned itself more with fashion as stronger perfumes became less necessary to combat stench as better hygiene took over and their association with the aristocracy became a sales barrier.

The use of perfumes became more closely associated with femininity when they were transferred from the pharmacy to the cosmetics counter, particularly with the emergence of Victorian-era ideas about distinct domains for men and women. The idea of a good smell in general was becoming more and more linked with the world of women, even though certain scents, like tobacco and pine, were still associated with masculinity.

While Europeans were more likely to bathe than Americans, the United States adopted innovative cleaning tools like toothbrushes and showers in the late 19th century, bolstered by the most recent hygiene research. Abundant space in the young nation of America also contributed to its clean regime. "Water mains and sewers were more easily installed in new cities than in ancient ones," Katherine Ashenburg writes in The Dirt on Clean. "Houses with bathrooms became the domestic norm, in contrast to Europe's old, crowded apartments."

An inventor in Philadelphia created the first popular commercial deodorant brand in 1888. It was given the moniker Mum, which translates to "keeping silent" or

"Mum's the word." Mum's first patented product was marketed as a waxy cream, which led to rapid imitations. However, these bulky products were difficult to apply and frequently left a greasy stain on clothes. Everdry invented the first antiperspirant in history in 1903; it blocked sweat pores by using aluminum chloride. Because these early antiperspirants were so strongly acidic, they too frequently caused clothing damage and stinging sensations for the wearer.

An inventor of Odo-Ro-No, an antiperspirant, wanted his hands to remain sweat-free during surgery early in the 1900s. To increase the company's sales, his daughter Edna Murphey hired an advertising agency in 1912. Their first popular advertisement presented excessive perspiration as a medical condition. A few years later, the company tried a different approach: persuading self-conscious women that no one would directly inform them about their body odor or B.O. for short. Soon, similar campaigns were launched against every conceivable imperfection, including bad breath, acne, torn stockings, gray hair, makeup flaws, and the ultimate — poor "feminine hygiene." The now-famous phrase "Often a bridesmaid, but never a bride" was created by Listerine, an oral antiseptic brand, to characterize the "life-destroying" effects of bad breath.

Due to their success in attracting female consumers, American deodorant companies started to subtly mention men's body odor in their advertisements by the 1930s. The first male-focused deodorant, Top-Flite, made its debut in 1935 and was sold in sleek black bottles. Other designs that were stereotypically associated with men followed, such as the Seaforth bottle that looked like a tiny whiskey jug. Ads for men's deodorant products frequently highlighted insecurities about money and implied that having an offensive body odor could harm one's career.

In the meantime, roll-on deodorant sticks, such as the 1940s applicator created by Mum employee Helen Diserens based on a ballpoint pen design, were replacing messy creams as the preferred method of delivery. Gillette released the first aerosol deodorant, Right Guard, at the beginning of the 1960s.

The abundance of deodorants, antiperspirants, soaps, colognes, perfumes, and douches that are available to us today all purport to mask bodily odors, even when those odors are the byproduct of physiological functions. "I think my favorite weird patent was based on baker's yeast," said Everts. "I just don't think I'd want to put baker's yeast in my armpit."

CHAPTER TWO

BODY ODOR: WHAT IS IT?

__NOTE THIS:__ Sweat doesn't directly cause body odor; rather, bacteria that live there cause it. Body odor can be controlled and avoided by taking action to stop perspiration from building up. It is a common misconception that sweat itself causes body odor. Human perspiration is actually nearly odorless. Body odor is the result of sweating people's skin bacteria breaking down sweat-containing protein molecules. While body odor is a common issue, it can negatively impact a person's quality of life. While personal hygiene habits are frequently the primary cause, body odor may occasionally be a sign of a more serious underlying medical issue. The mouth, other cavities, and bodily fluids can all produce odors *created by the body. On the other hand, the topic of this article is sweat bacteria and smells that come from the skin.*

The term "body odor" refers to any natural odor that comes from an individual. Odorants are a broad category of compounds that the human body is capable of producing. Many of these are essential for healthy bodily functions and do not produce offensive odors when present in small amounts. On the other hand, an excessive buildup of these substances on the skin may result in odors that are detectable.

Due to increased hormone activity and sweat gland activity during puberty, body odor typically becomes more noticeable during this period. Individuals who are obese or suffer from specific medical conditions, like diabetes, are also more prone to developing body odor. To humans, sweat itself has almost no smell. But foul odors can result from bacteria's quick growth and their breakdown of perspiration into acids. Therefore, those who perspire excessively, such as those who have hyperhidrosis, may be more prone to developing body odor.

The following locations are the most likely to experience body odor:

- Public and other hair

- The navel

- The anus

- In back of the ears

- The feet

- The groin

- The underarms

- The genitals

A person's particular body odor can be influenced by their food, natal sex, medical conditions, and medications. According to some research, animals are better than humans at recognizing each other by their unique scent profiles.

READ THIS ALSO ON WHAT BODY ODOUR IS: When sweat interacts with the bacteria on your skin, it produces an odor known as body odor. Perspiration doesn't smell by itself; rather, an odor is produced when perspiration and skin bacteria combine. Body odor can have an onion-like, tangy, sweet, or sour

smell. Your body odor is not always influenced by how much you sweat. For this reason, someone may not perspire but still have an offensive body odor. On the other hand, it is possible to perspire a lot but not smell. This is so because sweat alone does not cause body odor; rather, the type of bacteria on your skin and how those bacteria interact with perspiration do. Sweating is the fluid that your skin's surface secretes due to sweat glands. Sweat glands are classified as either apocrine or eccrine. The glands called apocrine are in charge of generating body odor.

ECCRINE GLANDS: Sweat is secreted directly onto your skin by eccrine glands. Sweat aids in cooling your skin and regulating body temperature as it evaporates. There is no scent released by it. Sweating causes your body temperature to rise, which can be counteracted by the cooling effect of sweat evaporating from your skin. Your palms and soles are among the majority of your body's eccrine glands.

APOCRINE GLANDS: Apocrine glands protrude into the follicles of your hair. The tube-like structure that holds your hair in your skin is called a hair follicle. Apocrine glands are located in the armpits and groin. When sweat from these glands comes into contact with bacteria on your skin, it releases an odor. Little children don't smell of body odor because apocrine glands don't function until puberty.

Although sweating is a normal bodily function, it can smell bad when it comes into contact with the skin because of certain foods, personal hygiene habits, or genetics. Variations in your sweating rate or body odor could be signs of a health problem.

WHAT ARE THE CAUSES OF BODY ODOR?

When sweat and bacteria on your skin come into contact, body odor results: Bacteria are found on our skin by nature. Odor can arise from the combination of bacteria, water, and fat found in sweat. There could be a strong, faint, or no smell at all. Body odor can be impacted by things like the foods you eat, hormones, or medications. Over sweating is a symptom of a condition known as hyperhidrosis. This condition may make people more prone to body odor due to excessive sweating, but sweaty palms and feet are typically most uncomfortable due to eccrine sweat glands. There's a chance that you'll smell bad every time you perspire. A bad body odor can affect some people more than others.

There are eccrine and apocrine sweat glands on an individual's skin. Apocrine glands are linked to hair follicles in the groin and underarms and begin to function during puberty. These glands secrete a thick, initially odorless sweat that is high in protein. However, body odor is caused by bacteria producing more odorant molecules in higher concentrations as they break down the abundance of proteins. Eccrine sweat glands, on the other hand, are primarily responsible for controlling body temperature through sweating and have less of an association with body odor.

Other elements that may influence body odor include:

- Work out.

- Anxiety or stress.

- Exposed to hot weather.

- Having a weight problem.

- Genetics.

CHAPTER THREE

COMMON TYPES OF BODY ODOR

Don't feel ashamed if you smell anywhere on your body; you're not the only one. For a multitude of reasons, it is normal to have odors in practically every part of the body. Schedule a consultation with a healthcare professional if the smell is strong or cannot be addressed with over-the-counter remedies.

SWEATING BENEATH THE ARMS: *What triggers it?* It's a basic fact of life that your underarms will smell. It's a normal process that results in an odor when perspiration, which is normally odorless, interacts with normal skin bacteria. The majority of sweat produced by apocrine glands, which are found in areas of the body with a lot of hair follicles like the armpit and groin, is produced in response to stress.

How do I go about fixing it? There are numerous strategies to get rid of underarm odors, like:

- Cleaning the vicinity

- Shaving the region since hair tends to retain smells

- Making use of deodorants or antiperspirants

- Dressing in absorbing clothes to keep sweat at bay

The effects of aluminum, which can be found in some antiperspirants, are a source of concern for medical professionals, and it's unclear whether exposure to high levels could have negative health effects. A select few decide to buy products devoid of aluminum.

FOUL BREATH: *Why does it occur?* Bad breath can be caused by a variety of factors, such as:

- Food particles lodged in the spaces between teeth

- Pathogens, including sinus infections

- Not using enough toothpaste or brushes

- Products made of tobacco

- Stones and tonsil infections

- Some GI disorders

- Specific lung infections

- Specific drugs

- Parched lips

- Infections of the gums and teeth

How do I go about fixing it? Frequently, improving oral hygiene can help treat foul breath. Additional typical fixes consist of:

- Using sugar-free gum to increase salivation

- Giving up cigarettes

- Making use of a tongue scraper

- Drinking less alcohol and coffee

- Sipping more water

- Using more brushes and floss

- Using mouthwash, particularly in the early morning and right before bed

Your need for a referral to a dentist or other specialist may depend on what is causing the odor.

ODOR OF URINE: *Why does it happen?* Urine can smell strange for a variety of reasons, such as:

- Lack of fluids

- Diabetes

- Infections of the urinary tract

- Coffee

- Foods heavy with sulfur

- Specific dietary supplements

How can I address this? If you detect a shift in the urine's smell:

- Consider consuming cranberry juice.

- Retain hydration

- Up your consumption of vitamin C

Consult a healthcare professional if you experience sudden or persistent changes in your urine that aren't related to your food or water intake.

SMELL OF FLATULENCE: *What triggers it?*

Although it's a normal and healthy bodily function to

pass gas, we could all do without the smell that goes along with it. It's possible that flatulence occasionally smells strongly and other times it doesn't. This is the reason: As food is broken down by our natural gut bacteria, sulfates are released. Food can accumulate sulfates, which results in an odor, if it remains in our intestines for an extended period of time. Stronger smells can also result from eating foods high in sulfur...

How do I go about fixing it? Since farts, including scented ones, are a natural part of the human experience, this one can be a little challenging. Having said that, if you're detecting overly potent smells, try:

- Steer clear of foods heavy in sulfur, like lentils, cabbage, and broccoli.

- Steer clear of foods that make you sick to your stomach or that you might be allergic to

- Examining probiotics

Speak with a healthcare professional if your flatulence is severe, such as if you're passing foul-smelling gas on a regular basis and you're also dealing with chronic abdominal pain, recurrent diarrhea or constipation, sudden weight changes, incontinence, or infection symptoms.

THE SMELL OF PENILE TISSUE: *Why does it occur?* There are numerous reasons why a person with a penis could smell something in their genital area.

- Urinary tract infection or UTI

- Fungal or yeast infection, which manifests as "jock itch"

- Stress (sweating is increased by apocrine glands in the groin when we are stressed)

- Balanitis or inflammation of the penis' head

- Smegma or a skin and oil accumulation around the penis

- STDs or sexually transmitted illnesses

How can I address this? Some of the problems might be resolved by using over-the-counter medications and practicing better genital hygiene. But since STIs and infections are frequently the source of genital odors, it's best to discuss your concerns with your doctor.

FOOT SMELL: *Why does it happen?* There are numerous reasons why feet smell, such as:

- Fungal infections of the skin, or athlete's foot

- Improperly drying your feet

- Consistently donning the same socks or shoes

How can I address this? Fortunately, there are lots of simple solutions to deal with foot odor, like:

- Maintaining dry feet

- Deodorizers for shoes

- Cream with antifungal properties

- Regularly changing socks

OUSTING VAGINA: *What leads to it?* Because there are numerous variations in the odors and causes of vaginal odors, determining their causes can be a little challenging. The most typical are as follows:

✓ **Tangy or fermented**: Lactobacilli are beneficial bacteria that are frequently found in the vagina. If the smell is sour, it is most likely the result of fermentation. An unpleasant stench resembling fermented food is more likely to occur in the presence of more of these bacteria.

✓ **Sweet and earthy:** Bacteria are probably the cause once more if you detect a smell that is sweet and earthy, like molasses! Vaginal pH fluctuates frequently, and there may occasionally be a faintly sweet smell.

✓ **Earthy and Smokey:** A musty smell may indicate stress. Stress causes our apocrine glands in the groin to produce more sweat.

✓ **Coppery:** Do your hands smell like that after handling change? Most likely, what you smell is copper, which is present in pennies. If you smell something coming from your vagina, it might be light bleeding after sex or menstrual blood, which contains iron and can smell metallic.

How can I address this? It is best to consult your healthcare provider about vaginal odors as the treatment for them will vary depending on the cause. This is particularly true if there is discharge along with the odor, since this could indicate a STI or infection.

ODOR FROM STOOL: *What triggers it?* And another unavoidable fact of life is poop. And the fact is, it stench most of the time. Our regular bacteria in our GI tracts and the foods we eat are to blame for this. But if you detect a particularly unpleasant smell coming from your poop, it could be because of:

- Intolerance to dairy

- Allergies to foods

- Pathogens

- A few drugs

How do I go about fixing it? It's best to speak with your healthcare provider about foul-smelling stool after you've tried avoiding foods that make you feel sick to your stomach. While generally unpleasant-smelling stool is normal and common, it is occasionally necessary to evaluate if the foul-smelling stool is indicative of malabsorption or another underlying medical issue.

CHAPTER FOUR

WHY SMELL OF SWEAT IS OFFENSIVE

Your sweat may smell bad for a number of reasons. For instance, certain foods, supplements, or medications may cause your sweat to smell bad. Recall that the smell comes from the bacteria on your skin interacting with the sweat, not from the sweat itself. A person's typical body odor can change due to a number of illnesses and medical conditions:

- Hyperactive thyroid

- Illness of the liver.

- Kidney disease.

- Illnesses caused by infections.

- Diabetes.

- Gout.

- Menopause

A change in body odor could indicate ketoacidosis associated with diabetes if you have the disease. Your blood becomes acidic and your body odor becomes fruity when your ketone levels are high. When you have liver or kidney disease, your body builds up toxins, which can make you smell like bleach.

FOOD ABLE TO PRODUCE BODY ODOR

It's possible that body odor is a result of diet. Consuming foods high in sulfur can cause body odor. It smells like rotten eggs, sulfur. Your body may release an unpleasant odor when it secretes it through perspiration. Foods high in sulfur include:

- Cabbage

- Broccoli

- Cauliflower

- Meat in red

- Onions

- Garlic

There are foods that increase perspiration. The additional perspiration may intensify your body odor. Although the foods don't directly cause body odor, they may have an impact on it because of how much they change perspiration patterns. Among them are:

- Monosodium glutamate (MSG)

- Coffee

- Spices like curry powder or cumin

- Hot sauce or other spicy food

- Alcohol

Body odor may be improved by getting rid of or minimizing these triggers.

CHAPTER FIVE

PREVENTING BODY ODOR

The groin and armpits have a high concentration of apocrine glands, which makes them vulnerable to the quick onset of body odor. But body odor can appear practically anywhere on the body. Despite the fact that there isn't a single cure for body odor, following these recommendations could help manage body odor:

APPLY AN ANTIPERSPIRANT OR DEODORANT:

Sweat is the bodily fluid through which waste products are expelled. Since we live in the tropical part of the world, one will produce more sweat, especially in the warmed parts of one's body, like the underarms and pubic region. The stench known as body odor is produced when bacteria react with this perspiration.

The correct deodorant can help reduce the smell of your body. Finding a deodorant that suits your body chemistry and daily needs may require some trial and error, but it's essential. Alcohol-based deodorants are frequently antibacterial, meaning they can temporarily eliminate bacteria before they cause an unpleasant odor on the body. According to medical professional Debra Wilson, deodorants are designed to get rid of underarm odor. They make your skin acidic when applied, which deters bacteria from liking it. Additionally, they typically include perfumes to cover up odors.

TAKE FREQUENT BATHS: Frequently, body odor is not caused by perspiration; rather, it results from the interaction of perspiration with bacteria on the skin. Showering at least once a day can help one stay clean by washing away perspiration and removing some bacteria from their skin. Dermatologist Stephanie Gardner claims that perspiration has no smell on its own. Gardner observed that sweat and skin bacteria combine to produce a strong odor and rapid bacterial growth. "Thorough washing, particularly in areas where you tend to perspire, can help prevent body odor," she stated.

MAKE SURE YOU THOROUGHLY DRY OFF: After taking a shower, thoroughly dry off, being especially mindful of any areas where you perspire a lot. It is more difficult for the bacteria that cause body odor to proliferate on dry skin.

GIVE UP DRINKING AND SMOKING: Due to the accumulation of toxins in the body, alcohol and smoking cause foul breath in addition to body odor. The odor of cigarettes clings to your body and clothes for a considerable amount of time. The liver can only metabolize roughly 12 ounces of beer per hour, according to substance abuse expert John Mayer, despite the fact that the body views alcohol as a toxin. He explained, "The body breaks down the remaining toxins into smaller parts called diacetic acid, carbon dioxide, and water that the body can metabolize and excrete through breath, sweat, and urine. This process is called oxidation.

However, drinking makes the blood vessels close to the skin enlarge, making people feel hot and consequently causing the body to sweat and, frequently, produce body odor. This could explain why perspiration is more obvious.

ELIMINATE FABRIC SOFTENERS: Fabric softeners are typically used by most people when doing laundry. When washing clothes, a liquid called a fabric softener is used to lessen wrinkles and soften the fabric. Nevertheless, body odor may result from fabric softeners because they cling to the fibers of clothing, obstructing airflow and evaporating. As beneficial as fabric softeners are, Wilson stated that improper management of them can result in this side effect. They may hinder your ability to breathe and keep bacteria that cause odors at bay. Detergent's ability to penetrate fibers and eliminate perspiration, bacteria, and body odors is also hindered. It is possible for softeners to irritate skin.

MAKE USE OF ANTIBACTERIAL SOAP: Some odor-causing bacteria can be eliminated by giving you a thorough bath with an antibacterial soap bar. Antibacterial soaps have the ability to target the bacteria on the body, thereby reducing their offensive odor. "You can consult a dermatologist to select an antibacterial soap that is appropriate for your skin type, ensuring that you do not develop any skin allergies or infections after using the antibacterial soap," Wilson stated.

GIVE YOUR UNDERARMS A SHAVE: Although shaving your underarms won't stop you from perspiring, it might help you stay away from stinky areas. Because hair is porous, perspiration-induced odors are absorbed by it. Having too much hair makes a swampy area that can harbor bacteria and cause you to smell bad. Additionally, an excess of hair slows down the evaporation process by trapping moisture. "Just grab your razor and shave it off to avoid all the fuss," stated Gardner. It will minimize bacteria and give you a more youthful feeling, so reducing the odor. After engaging in any physical activity, change your clothes and give your underarms a wash for additional care.

FREQUENTLY CHANGE YOUR CLOTHES: After a day out or even after working out, it can be tempting to rewear the same outfits. This is not recommended because odor-causing bacteria love these kinds of environments. It is best to change into fresh clothes after a demanding workday and to remove perspiring workout attire as soon as you finish exercising. "Change your clothes often when you are sweating heavily," Gardner advised. Wearing clean clothing reduces body odor. Be sure to change your socks as well, especially if you tend to have foot odor. Go barefoot whenever you can, change your insoles frequently, and use deodorant powders in your shoes.

Your body odor is a direct result of what you eat. Broccoli, cauliflower, and cabbage are examples of foods high in sulfur that can change your smell. Odor-causing food ingredients include onions, garlic, curries, and other strong spices. "Be mindful of what you eat," Wilson advised. Eat less or avoid foods that could give off odors. Foods that tend to increase perspiration, like spicy or hot peppers, can also cause an unpleasant odor on your body. Odor-causing bacteria can proliferate in your sweat due to the scent of foods like onions and garlic.

MODIFY YOUR LAUNDRY ROUTINE: Body odor can start to affect how your clothes smell after several wears. By using these modern laundry tips and tricks, you can prevent odor-causing clothing:

- Quickly wash perspiring apparel. The stench will be harder to remove from your clothing the longer you wait.

- Garment clothes from the inside out. Since your clothes are most affected on the inside, the detergent will remove sweat and odor from there more effectively.

- To your laundry cycle, add one cup of distilled white vinegar. Tough, lingering smells will be lessened with this. Alternatively, you could choose to add ½ cup of baking soda to your laundry load (do not mix the two).

- Apply some laundry sanitizer. Eliminating the bacteria present in your clothing with laundry sanitizer can potentially lessen the smell.

- Ditch the dryer or dry on cool. Your clothes' stench may get worse from warm, musty dryers. Attempt air drying your clothing or using a cool setting in the dryer.

PUT ON BREEZY ATTIRE: Wearing natural fibers like cotton and jute is another golden rule, particularly for hot climates. Steer clear of tight clothing and synthetic clothing that restricts airflow to the skin. Put on airy, loose clothing that will allow air to circulate and keep you cool. "Though sweating is good for your health because it releases toxins through your skin, it can also cause uncomfortable sweat patches that can occasionally be embarrassing," Gardner stated. Choose airy clothing with natural fibers to prevent situations like this and allow your skin to breathe. Your perspiration increases when you wear a garment that retains it, which aggravates and discomforts you even more. Pick materials like cotton, light wool, and linen. They prevent perspiration and the development of body odor because they have moisture-absorbing qualities and allow air to pass through.

UTILIZE NATURAL SOLUTIONS: If you feel like your deodorant needs a little extra help, try applying or cleaning smelly areas with natural antibacterial like baking soda, witch hazel, lemon juice, apple cider vinegar, or tea tree oil. The antiseptic qualities of these DIY kitchen and medicine cabinet remedies eliminate excess bacteria and restore equilibrium to your skin's pH level.

Apply the mixture to dry, clean skin by wetting a cotton ball with your preferred ingredient. Use sparingly after combining one part baking soda with one part water to create a paste. You could also decide to apply a half-lemon rub to the afflicted areas. Steer clear of any areas that might be burned, scraped, or cut. It is best to stay away from ingredients like baking soda, tea tree oil, and apple cider vinegar if you have sensitive skin because they can irritate it. Rather, apply a cotton ball soaked in a mixture of equal parts water and lemon juice to the skin.

CHANGES IN HORMONES CAUSE BODY ODOR

Certainly, hormonal fluctuations can give you a smelly body. Changes in body odor are caused by excessive sweating, which is a result of hot flashes, night sweats, and hormonal fluctuations during menopause. Certain people think that menstruation or pregnancy cause changes in body odor. Ovulation, the point in a woman's menstrual cycle when she can become pregnant, is thought to be when her body odor changes in an attempt to attract a mate.

DIAGNOSIS OF BODY ODOR

Your doctor will probably perform an examination and inquire about your medical history in order to diagnose a problem with sweating and body odor. Your blood or urine may be tested by the doctor. The tests can determine whether an infection, diabetes, or hyperthyroidism—an overactive thyroid—is the source of your issue.

PROVEN TREATMENT OF BODY ODOR

Your healthcare provider can identify the underlying cause of your excessive sweating and body odor through physical examination, blood, or urine testing. Treatments for these conditions are based on this information. Using a deodorant or antiperspirant could be a straightforward solution if you're worried about perspiration and body odor.

ANTIPERSPIRANT: Antiperspirants contain substances derived from aluminum that temporarily obstruct sweat pores, lowering the quantity of sweat that reaches your skin.

ALUMINUM CHLORIDE: Antiperspirants with prescriptions that contain aluminum chloride may be suggested by a physician or dermatologist. When aluminum chloride is absorbed through the skin, it lessens perspiration. 10% to 30%Trusted Source aluminum chloride may be present in prescription antiperspirants.

BOTULINUM TOXIN: For those who perspire excessively, a doctor may prescribe Botox treatment. In order to prevent the release of chemicals that cause sweating, they might inject Botox directly into the skin. Per certain reports, 82–87% less sweating is reported after receiving Botox injections under the arms.

DEODORANTS: Sweat cannot be removed by deodorants, but odor can. They usually contain alcohol and make your skin acidic, which deters bacteria from growing on it. Perfume scents are frequently added to deodorants in an effort to cover up odors.

PRESCRIPTION MEDICINES MAY PREVENT SWEATING: Your healthcare professional will advise you to use caution if they recommend this because your body needs to sweat in order to cool itself when necessary.

SURGERY: An endoscopic thoracic sympathectomy (ETS) is a procedure that a doctor can do if self-care and medication are not sufficient to treat severe body odor. This cuts off the nerves that regulate perspiration beneath the armpit skin. This is a last resort that carries the risk of damaging nearby arteries and other nerves. Nonetheless, a 2019 review discovered that after undergoing ETS, over 90% of patients reported having a higher quality of life.

CHAPTER SIX

LIFESTYLE AND PERSONAL HYGIENE (SELF-HELP)

There are several DIY methods you can use to lessen perspiration and body odor. The ideas listed below could be beneficial:

TAKE A DAILY BATH: Frequent bathing inhibits the growth of bacteria on your skin, especially when using antibacterial soap. By using antibacterial soap in your daily bath or shower, you can keep your skin clean. Pay attention to the areas, such as your armpits and groin, where you perspire the most. Unpleasant body odor can be avoided by routinely eliminating some of the bacteria on your skin.

CHOOSE CLOTHING TO SUIT YOUR ACTIVITY:

Select natural materials for everyday clothing, such as silk, wool, and cotton. Your skin can breathe thanks to these. You might prefer synthetic clothing made to wick moisture away from your skin when working out. Put on cotton clothing that fits loosely. This permits airflow to your skin. Bras and undergarments fall under this rule as well. Clothing made of moisture-wicking material, which can draw moisture away from the skin, is also beneficial.

TRY PRACTICING SOME RELAXATION METHODS:

Consider relaxation techniques, such as yoga, meditation or biofeedback. Through these exercises, you can learn to manage the stress that leads to perspiration. Look for strategies to lessen your stress.

Your apocrine glands may become active when you are stressed.

MODIFY YOUR FOOD HABITS: You may perspire more than usual or notice a stronger than usual body odor if you consume caffeinated beverages and spicy or strongly scented foods. It might be helpful to avoid these foods. Consider cutting out particularly odorous foods from your diet or observe whether certain foods exacerbate body odor. Foods like alcohol, garlic, and onions can all intensify the odor of perspiration.

APPLY A TOPICAL ANTIPERSPIRANT; it functions by attracting perspiration back into the sweat glands. Your body sends a signal that your sweat glands are full, which causes your sweat production to decrease.

These consist of both prescription and over-the-counter deodorants.

SHAVE YOUR ARMPITS to ensure that perspiration evaporates fast and has less time to interact with bacteria. Hair serves as a haven for bacteria. And also wash your clothes frequently, and make sure they are clean.

BEST DEODORANT FOR SMELLING ARMPITS

Deodorants function by disguising body odor with a more enticing scent. Conversely, antiperspirants lessen your perspiration. Make sure the product you use under your arms says "antiperspirant" on the label. Aluminum is the main component of most antiperspirants. Before going to bed and after taking a bath or shower, apply antiperspirant. For the best effects, apply antiperspirants to dry skin. Your healthcare provider may be able to prescribe a stronger antiperspirant if over-the-counter options are ineffective.

CHAPTER SIX

ELIMINATE BODY ODOR NATURALLY

There might be effective solutions if you'd like to treat underarm body odor in a more natural way. Consult your healthcare provider regarding:

APPLE CIDER VINEGAR: Fill a spray bottle with a small amount of water and apple cider vinegar. Apply the blend under your arms. Bacteria are killed by the acid in vinegar. It offers a long and impressive list of health advantages. It relieves acid reflux and heartburn, helps eliminate toxins, controls blood sugar, and even promotes weight loss.

In addition to its astringent properties, vinegar helps eliminate bacteria and constrict pores when applied topically to the skin. If you perspire a lot, putting a vinegar mixture topically or drinking it every night can help minimize perspiration. Before breakfast, lunch and dinner, take a concoction of one teaspoon of apple cider vinegar and two teaspoons of vinegar. It should start to dry out in a few days or so.

LEMON JUICE: Shake well with a mixture of lemon juice and water. Mist the concoction beneath your arms. The citric acid in lemon juice kills bacteria. Lemons are an excellent natural remedy for reducing excessive perspiration because of their acidic content. You can either use a cotton pad to apply a small amount of lemon juice and baking soda, or you can rub half a lemon on your underarms, gently pressing to release the liquid. After rinsing well, try to leave the lemon juice on for at least half an hour.

BAKING SODA AND CORNSTARCH: Use water and baking soda to make a paste. After applying the paste to your armpits, allow it to dry. Both smells and the acidity of your skin are balanced by baking soda. Natural water-absorbing substances are cornstarch and baking soda. As an all-natural deodorant, baking soda works by neutralizing the acids that sweat contains that are conducive to bacterial growth. For this reason, baking soda is an ingredient in a lot of store-bought deodorants!

When applying a thick mixture of the two directly to the sweaty area of your underarms each night, make sure they are completely dry. Before giving it a quick water rinse, let it sit for half an hour. I should warn you that if you leave the mixture on for too long, uncomfortable side effects may occur. My skin became irritated and my armpits turned a bright red when I tried this about a year ago and left the baking soda on all day. This hack did not work for me again because the baking soda also caused a burning sensation.

JUICE FROM TOMATOES: Tomato juice has anti-cancer properties, but it also reduces chronic sweating and pores. You can manage excessive perspiration by eating a diet high in tomatoes or just by consuming a glass of tomato juice every day. Try applying tomato juice to your underarms or any other area where you sweat a lot and letting it sit there for at least ten minutes before washing it off if you're not a fan of tomatoes.

ETHERMOUTH COCONUT OIL: Sweat and odor are among the many ailments that coconut oil seems to be able to cure these days. This is because the superfruit have lauric acid, an antimicrobial that destroys bacteria that cause perspiration. Here's how to use coconut oil to reduce offensive odor and excessive sweating:

- Mix one cup coconut oil with ten grams of crushed camphor.

- Combine the ingredients, and then apply the mixture to your body.

- Let it sit on your skin for half an hour to an hour.

- Use water to rinse it off.

As you would with a typical moisturizer, you can also massage cold-pressed coconut oil into your skin right after taking a shower or bath. Do this regularly to decrease excessive sweat.

GREEN/BLACK TEA: To make green tea, immerse tea bags in warm water. Spend a few minutes each day under your armpits with the soaked tea bags in place. Green tea might help stop sweating by clogging your pores. Tea and other hot beverages seem to go against the idea of preventing perspiration. However, the magnesium and vitamin B in green tea constrict sweat glands and promote calmness, so say goodbye to sweating under pressure!

To benefit from these sweat-blocking properties, consider substituting green tea for your morning coffee if you perspire excessively. When applied directly to the skin, black tea's astringent qualities can help minimize perspiration if you suffer from persistent underarm sweating. Use a towel or the tea bag itself to rub the black tea on your underarms for a few minutes after brewing and letting it cool.

JUICE MADE FROM WHEATGRASS: Wheatgrass juice, a natural detoxifier, is high in folic acid, vitamin A, C, B12, and B6. All it takes to combat sweat is one tablespoon of wheatgrass per day to neutralize and dilute blood toxins. You're in luck if the odor emanating from your sweat is strong! Sweat odor is also lessened by wheatgrass juice.

OIL FROM TEA TREES: Tea tree oil works as an astringent to combat bacteria that cause perspiration, just like tea and vinegar do. Every day, blot your underarms with a cotton ball soaked in tea tree oil. The effects should start to show in a few days.

POTATOES AND ADDITIVES RICH IN POTASSIUM: Your body will retain more water if you eat too much sodium. Potatoes and broccoli, which are high in potassium, help the body expel water by reversing this process. Potatoes are known to absorb excess water as a result of this reaction, which also helps to reduce sweating. To get these drying effects, just rub a potato slice across your armpits for a few minutes every day.

HAZEL WITCH: For perspiring underarms, witch hazel is an excellent DIY treatment. Witch hazel is an astringent and an antiperspirant that is found in nature. It eliminates perspiration by drying out your skin and sealing your pores.

Applying liquid witch hazel to the areas where you perspire the most using a cotton ball is the first step. Another way to create a paste is to mix equal parts water and powdered hazel bark. After rubbing the paste onto your skin, rinse it off with water after an hour. Witch hazel is a remedy that can be used as an astringent for your face, to remove makeup, or even to treat dandruff, even though it's unlikely that you have any in your medications.

WHITE POWDER FOR SANDALWOOD: Powdered white sandalwood is an additional natural astringent. To make a home remedy for hyperhidrosis, mix one tablespoon each of lemon juice, rose water, and white sandalwood powder. Blend the mixture until a paste is formed. Apply the paste to your skin after giving it a thorough wash and drying. Make sure to allow it to solidify entirely. Use warm water to rinse your skin after 20 to 30 minutes. To lessen perspiration, repeat this procedure each day.

USE SALT: Dryer pits with salt? Indeed, I say. Your skin stays dry, your pores are blocked, and sweat is absorbed by salt.

As a homemade treatment for hyperhidrosis, you have two choices. To start, apply sea salt crystals to the areas of your body that perspire. To use whenever you sense a sweat session starting, you can even keep a bottle of crystals with you. If you still have trouble, try making a citrus scrub by mixing equal parts lime juice and salt.

Enjoy sweating less after rubbing the solution onto your skin and rinsing it off.

WHEN TO MAKE A DOCTOR'S APPOINTMENT

Which body odor and sweating symptoms should worry you? If you encounter any of the following symptoms, think about getting in touch with your healthcare provider:

- Often perspiring or wearing clothes drenched in perspiration, even when not moving or in a warm environment.

- Sweating so much that it interferes with daily activities such as trying to hold a pen, turn a doorknob or use a computer.

- Perspiring when you're asleep

- Sweat constantly dampening the skin.

- Frequent skin infections in body areas prone to sweating.

- A sweet body odor, which can be a sign of diabetes

- A bleach-like body odor, which could be a sign of liver or kidney disease

- An abrupt shift in body odor or an increase in perspiration

CHAPTER SEVEN

IN SUMMARY

Body odor is a common problem that is frequently treated at home. It is not caused by the smell of perspiration; rather, it is a consequence of bacteria breaking down proteins in a person's sweat. It's not always the case that body odor is associated with offensive odors, despite the common misconception.

Using antiperspirants, shaving, and thorough washing can all help someone manage unpleasant body odor. A physician might suggest prescription medications and, in certain situations, surgery if symptoms don't go away. Sweating excessively and body odor could also be signs of an underlying medical issue. A person should see a doctor right away if they notice any sudden changes in the amount of sweat they produce or their body odor.

FAQs ABOUT BODY ODOR

It can be difficult for many of us to discuss the odors our bodies produce. However, it's normal to have questions about them because they're an inherent part of life. Here we address some frequently asked questions concerning body odors, such as what causes them and whether they should raise red flags.

WHAT IS BODY ODOR? Any smell emanating from a human is referred to as "body odor." Our bodies actually produce odors in many different places, despite the fact that most people associate body odor with sweat. Many different compounds, referred to as odorants, are produced by the human body. Numerous of these compounds are essential for various body processes, but when they build up together, they can produce odors that are both noticeable and frequently bad.

Ordinarily treatable at home, body odor is a common concern that should not be taken too seriously. A person's quality of life may be negatively impacted by an offensive stench if it is ignored. Additionally, certain odors that are bothersome or persistent may be signs of a medical issue that needs to be addressed.

HOW CAN I DISCUSS BODY ODOR WITH MY PHYSICIAN? Temporary body odors are generally acceptable. On the other hand, bodily odor can occasionally reveal information about our health. If your overall health changes at the same time as you notice a change in body odor that lasts longer than a few weeks, you should consult your physician.

It's not appropriate to feel ashamed of body odor; doctors have seen and heard it all. Trust us. Whenever you talk to your provider about a body odor, try to be as specific and direct as you can. This will enable them to precisely identify the source of your body odor and the most effective course of action.

WHY IS THE AREA UNDER MY ARMS THE ONLY PART OF MY BODY THAT SMELLS? The groin and armpits are the primary locations for apocrine sweat glands. The Apocrine sweat glands generate a solution that includes proteins and pheromones, while the majority of sweat glands excrete a solution that is 99%

water. Sweaty armpits smell because odor-producing bacteria eat this protein. Use a flannel or sponge to wash these areas instead of just your hands because their rougher texture will collect more bacteria and provide a deeper clean.

WHY DOES MY PERSPIRATION HAVE A STRONGER SMELL THAN MOST PEOPLE'S?

Increased perspiration increases the likelihood of developing body odor. Sweat will smell stronger if it builds up from not washing or from wearing dirty clothes, but there are other things that can make your body smell worse:

- ✓ **Diet:** Spicy and pungent foods will cause you to perspire and may give off an overpowering odor when you sweat. Additionally, a lot of strong foods contain oils that permeate your skin and then into your blood.

- ✓ **Genetics:** Because they have more sweat glands and produce more protein, some people will naturally sweat more than others. Sweating more than usual can also be a sign of a thyroid condition.

- ✓ You'll perspire more when you exercise, are anxious, or overweight.

HOW CAN I GET RID OF BODY ODOR?

- ✓ Wash your hands every day. If you already wash your hands, use an antibacterial soap to help eliminate the bacteria that cause odors. Goods like Cuticura, Valderma, or anything from the Australian Tea Tree line which includes a nice assortment of all-natural, antibacterial body, face, and hair washes are appropriate. Give the groin and armpits extra attention when using an antibacterial cleanser.

✓ Use antiperspirant products like Driclor, Perspirex, or Odaban to lessen sweating.

✓ Freshen up: Use a perfume or body spray to cover up any odors.

✓ Clean clothes: Only use fresh towels and linens, and put on clean clothes each morning.